LOVING THOSE WITH
FIBRO

Caring for those with the invisible disease.

Michael R. Holien

Cover Art by Stacy Ihlenfeld

Cover Design by Peter J. Epler

Back Cover Photo by Kristen Proby Photography

Printed in the United States of America

ISBN-13: 978-1499294231

ISBN-10: 1499294239

First Edition

For my sweet wife, April, and the men and women who struggle with Fibromyalgia daily.

You are my heroes.

~M.

CONTENTS

INTRODUCTION

In the early part of 2014, I sat down and wrote what you are about to read. I have been writing all of my adult life, and I have never struggled with writing like I have struggled writing "Loving Those With Fibro". The disease of Fibromyalgia has entered the life of my family through my dear wife April, and it has attempted to destroy us, but we refuse to lie down in defeat. We choose to fight back with the mightiest weapon we can find… hope. We choose hope over despair. We choose hope over destruction. We choose hope over defeat. We CHOOSE hope. If this little book can bring you hope and awareness about Fibromyalgia, then the work that went into it will have been worth it.

Now, please understand: I am not a doctor of any kind. I am not a counselor, psychologist/psychiatrist, nutritionist, life coach or a physical therapist. Neither do I speak from ANY professional platform or education. I am just a guy. Well I am more than that. I am a husband who loves his wife, who struggles everyday with an illness that cannot be seen outside the pain I see in her beautiful face. This little book is not to give advice other than some helpful tips on how to approach a loved one who struggles with Fibro.

And perhaps I wish to share with some of my Fibro friends some words of hope:

You are loved.

You are not alone.

You can find peace in this life.

We are all in this together.

~M

"Elen sila lumenn' omentielvo, a star shines on the hour of our meeting."

~ J.R.R. Tolkien,

The Fellowship of the Ring

GREETINGS

Hello. My name is Mike, and I am married to the most spectacular woman on planet Earth. (Sorry guys; she's taken.) I adore my wife to the very core, but there is something I want you to know about her. My beautiful, smart, intelligent, godly, fun and spirited wife has a disease called Fibromyalgia (henceforth, "Fibro"). If you are not familiar with this disease, you may not know that it plagues six million people in the United States today. You may not know that people who have Fibro have a myriad of different symptoms including, but not limited to: muscle pain and fatigue, trouble sleeping, morning stiffness, headaches, painful menstrual periods, tingling or numbness in hands and feet, and problems with thinking/memory (sometimes called "fibro fog").*

Again, if you are unfamiliar with this disease, you may not know that for all the world's vast medical knowledge, no one really knows what causes it. So, for six million people in the US alone, there is a very present reality of knowing they will face constant physical pain every day. Sounds crappy, huh? Well, in many ways it is, but did you know that there is something you can do so your friends and loved ones who suffer with Fibro can actually live fulfilling and rewarding lives in the midst of their struggle?

Yes, you can! And I want to help you know what that is, but first, a little about mine and April's story. I met April when she was just a girl. Okay, she was 18, but still very young and I must admit that when I met her, I was enamored. April was (and is) beautiful, independent, godly, funny, and spirited. Notice that the last word has been underlined for emphasis. I mean, when I met April, I pretty much knew she was the one for me, SO at the ripe old age of 21, I pursued and dated and wooed this precious gem. Eight months later, before a mass of family and friends, April and I were wed in our home church and so began our life's journey together.

And the journey was a blast.

At that time in our lives, we had four red haired little kids, a great career in ministry, and we were living in the most beautiful place imaginable! We were living the dream. Then one day, we woke up to a day that was unlike any other we had ever experienced before. On this particular day, it was as if someone had flipped a switch in April's body. All of a sudden she was in excruciating pain and extremely tired. Well, she was tired during the day, but unfortunately not at night. So sleeping at night stopped, and I became worried.

After a battery of tests and an array of blood samples, MRIs, and consultations from wise doctors, we were given the news that my wife was suffering with Fibromyalgia, a disease I had never previously heard of in my life.

After doing due diligence with Google and Wikipedia I came to some personal conclusions. Thinking that ten minutes of reading online made me an expert, I spoke loudly and arrogantly my opinions of the doctors on this disease. These statements only hurt my wife and caused her more pain than the disease itself. (I never said I was all that bright.)

But friends, my family and I have lived with this disease for over four years now. April has continued to fight most courageously, and after I have had years to ponder and to experience this in my own family, I am now comfortable sharing some advice to you as you approach someone who suffers from Fibro.

You can be an instrument of HOPE for your loved one by doing some simple things…

"If you judge people, you have no time to love them."

~Unknown

JUDGMENTS

1. **DON'T** make judgments and air your opinions about the disease of Fibromyalgia.

If you are one of the people who don't believe Fibro is a real thing, don't tell someone who suffers with it, "It's all in your head." The medical community has done a lot of research on Fibro and has concluded that it is a real disease; they just haven't been able to find the cause of it. Many people get confused and think that if a cause cannot be found, then it is not a real disease. Fibro is real and your loved one is truly suffering. To tell him or her that it is all in their head, like I ashamedly admit to having done, is degrading and cruel. Instead…

DO admit that you don't know much about the disease. Tell your friend that although Fibro isn't a disease that you are familiar with, you are willing to learn more about it. Most of all, tell him or her that you will not abandon them as they journey toward wellness. Your Fibro-suffering friends need to know you care and that they are not alone.

Questions to Consider:

What are some ways you can educate yourself about Fibromyalgia?

_____

_____

_____

After you learn some things, write them down here for a quick reminder:

_____

_____

_____

_____

"Don't walk behind me; I may not lead. Don't walk in front of me; I may not follow. Just walk beside me and be my friend."

~Albert Camus

2. **DON'T** stop asking him or her to "do stuff" with you. When I met my wife she was a mover and groover. She loved to be out and about and to socialize with friends and family all the time, but since she has been suffering with the Fibro fog and chronic pain, she finds it difficult to be as active as she once was. In fact, she often finds it impossible. Because she has to decline so many invitations, people often think she does not want to go out. Nothing is farther from the truth. She loves her family and friends, and often grieves that she cannot take part; however, she still likes to be asked. Why? Because Fibro people still want to be included, even if it's a smaller part. So…

DO keep inviting your friend to experience life with you! Send emails, make calls and do not stop stamping out cards, because even if you receive an "I'm sorry but…" reply, you are encouraging your friend with kind words. Your notes say, "I'm still here and still want you in my life." If you really want to go the extra mile to involve your friend, find ways to modify your activity so that your Fibro friend can participate. A few months ago, April told me that she was sorry that our two younger children didn't have the active mom that the older kids had. She was grieved that she couldn't make all the open houses, Valentines parties, and such. Instead of just patting her on the back and saying "there, there", I decided to create ways that she could participate more with the little ones. One big thing that we did was to re-institute (and make mandatory) a weekly dinner at the table. I know what you're thinking: "Didn't we always eat at the table in our day?" Yes, we did, but times have changed. Now we have become SO busy that a lot of times we eat on the run. So by reestablishing this practice in our home, we enjoy "being" together. It has been a huge success. How might a good friend change some activities to include a Fibro friend?

-Instead of inviting him or her to the gym to run laps, offer to come over and walk around the block.

-Instead of inviting him or her to the coffee house, bring over a carafe of some fine coffee and share a cup.

-Instead of inviting him or her to your church for Sunday school class, perhaps offer to start a small study with them at their home.

-Instead of inviting your buddy to go out hunting, offer to bring over a hunting video and some steaks to grill.

-Instead of inviting your gal pal to go out to the spa, offer to bring over your nail polish collection and give her a mani-pedi. (Yes, my wife has my man card. Why do you ask?)

You get the point. Doing stuff together is about being together right? Just change up what you do, and you will be a blessing to your friend.

Questions to Consider:

Remember you know your Fibro friend better than anyone! Can you think of some other ways to include your friend?

_____

_____

_____

_____

_____

_____

Name one thing you could try this week:

_____

"I do not at all understand the mystery of grace -
only that it meets us where we are but does not
leave us where it found us."

~Anne Lamott

3. **DON'T** make your Fibro friend feel bad if they have to back out or change plans at the last second. This is especially important for spouses! Here is the scenario: your spouse actually slept a whole seven hours last night! Woohoo! You bring coffee and he/she rolls out of bed with a smile. As the day progresses, you see they're having a rather good day. No complaints about pain- they are at the sink doing dishes, and so you go for it: "How about date night tonight?" They smile at you and reply, "That sound great! Let's go see that new movie."

You feel great! Boom! You may even aim to take him or her out for dinner, but 4:00 pm comes around and your loved one gets a flare up. They "med up" and are down for the count, so it's Netflix and some microwave popcorn on the couch. Sound familiar? Yes. Disappointing? Uh, yes. Your spouse's fault? No. No, no, no! It's the stinking Fibro's fault. A wise man once said, "Be mad at Fibro, not at your spouse." Good words.

So when plans inevitably change...

DO understand and cut him or her some slack. At our house we call this grace. Instead of using words of discouragement, voice that although you ARE discouraged, you understand and can reschedule for another time. You can also make room on the couch and pop two bags of popcorn and watch Netflix together. This may not be ideal for you, but again, being together was the main point of date night, right?

One day some people from our church offered to keep our kids for the night so we could go out to dinner and a movie. What a blessing!! I could tell as the day progressed, however, that the "going out" option was diminishing. So did I cancel the sitter and sulk in the cab of my truck? HECK, NO! We dropped of the kids, hit the grocery store and picked up steaks and crab-stuffed mushrooms, and I mashed taters at home. We pigged out on food and a million episodes of our favorite TV show. It was an epic night, and we had a blast.

Questions to Consider:

What are some ways that you have been disappointed because of changed plans due to a flare up?

_____

_____

_____

_____

_____

How did you react/what did you end up doing instead?

_____

_____

_____

_____

_____

What are some ways you can be proactive for next time?

_____

_____

_____

_____

_____

"Against the assault of laughter nothing can stand."
~ Mark Twain

"Life is worth living as long as there's a laugh in it."
~L.M. Montgomery,
Anne of Green Gables

4. **DON'T** forget to laugh. If you were to ask five of my closest friends what my top quality was, you would not hear, "Mike sure is intelligent." Although I am smart, it's not my top quality, and probably not why people like me, but I do like to laugh, and laugh and laugh and laugh. I love good jokes, and pranks and funny situations, and most of all I love to laugh with my wife. We have fun together, but something happens when you live with a life altering disease: you forget to laugh, and you focus on the stuff that stinks. I know April and I do that from time to time. Sometimes being friends with a Fibro sufferer can be difficult. When they suffer, you tend to suffer. The laughs can get less and less, but you don't have to let that happen!

DO find things to laugh about so you won't lose the sparkle in your friendship, but you may be asking, "How do I laugh in situations that are un-laughable?" The answer is that you look for the funny through the pain. Allow me to set the scene: On particularly high pain days, Fibro patients "med up". In case you do not know what this term means, let me fill you in. Many Fibro patients take several different prescription drugs to help them cope with their symptoms. On days when they cannot sleep, they take sleeping pills. On days when their muscles are so cramped they cannot stand it, they take a muscle relaxer. On extreme pain days, when the pain is so bad that all they can do is cry, they take both over the counter and prescription pain medication. On the *really* bad flare up days, when they get the trifecta of all calamities, they take all three (or more) of their meds. Most of the time only their closest friends know about this. You know- their spouses and kids and besties... because in America there is a bias against people who take pain meds as if they were some sort of "crack addict" and as if this makes him or her a bad person. No kidding; we have heard it all, but there are days when a Fibro friend needs to "med up" to care for themselves. So how is this funny? On occasion, April and I will have a good laugh that she, a pastor's wife, after taking her duly prescribed meds, gets a bit "chatty". April ordinarily is very sweet and funny and kind, but when she is on meds, she is sweet and funny and kind... times ten! We laugh because of the situation we find ourselves in. We laugh because little things just seem funnier when you're medicated. We laugh because we share a deep love and bond for one another. We laugh because on many days we would cry if we did not laugh, and would not we rather laugh?

Keep laughing. Watch funny movies. Retell the awesome stories that you shared with your friend. Laugh!

Questions to Consider:

Do you find it hard to laugh in your struggles?

_____

What are some ways you can bring the joy of laughter back into your life?

_____

_____

_____

_____

Name five activities you can do to help you laugh more:

_____

_____

_____

_____

_____

"Hope

Smiles from the threshold of the year to come,

Whispering 'it will be happier'..."

~Alfred Tennyson

5. **DON'T** ever give up hope for your friend. EVER. I have a friend named Joe Coco who is very wise. One day he said to me, "Mike, humankind needs hope. Without it we perish." If there is something your Fibro friend needs more than anything else right now, it is hope. Now, hear me: I am not saying that you should inundate your friend with a hundred different books, articles and web sites telling him or her how to "cure" Fibro. Your friend does not need that. They read more books, articles and web sites than you can possibly imagine. My wife rarely goes to sleep before 3 am. *Every day.* She spends much of her time reading. She doesn't need me bringing her homework every time I come home from work. Never giving up hope for him or her means not becoming negative and start saying things like, "Just get over it and learn to live with it." That would be like me dousing you with gasoline, lighting you on fire and saying, "Just deal with it bro; it's the way it is," and although I know this analogy breaks down because you're not the one that gave your friend Fibro, it still points to the cruelty of our words when you do not consider them thoroughly. The truth is that there IS reason for hope. In the past year there has been a medical break-through on Fibro (check out this article: http://www.medicaldaily.com/breakthrough-

fibromyalgia-research-pain-your-skin-not-your-head-246925). Every day medical researchers make advances against various diseases, and it is helpful, optimistic, and healthy to hope that Fibromyalgia might be the next one on the list to be conquered.

DO offer words of hope to your friend daily, words like "I love you... I believe good days are ahead... I know you can do this... I think you just might be the most awesome person I know... You inspire me... We're gonna kick Fibro's butt together... I know that today kinda stinks, but tomorrow might be the best day of your life!" Words of hope may seem like a small thing to you, but each of us needs to believe that the best days are ahead. Fibro friends need hope, and they can find it in you.

Questions to Consider:

How can you inspire your Fibro friend today?

_____

_____

_____

_____

What gifts and skills do you have that your friend needs?

_____

_____

Pick one of these ways to bless your Fibro friend today:

-Send a card.

-Clean their cat box. (Seriously)

-Deliver some flowers.

-Fix a delicious lunch and share it.

-Do wash their dishes.

"People can tell you to keep your mouth shut, but that doesn't stop you from having your own opinion."

~Anne Frank,

The Diary of a Young Girl

MY TWO BITS

If you are reading this today and you or a loved one who suffers with Fibromyalgia (or any chronic pain or disability, for that matter) I want you to know that you are not alone. You have April and me. We get you. We understand that life has changed and that it is difficult. We understand that the day-to-day grind of suffering and setback gets old, and that you might feel like throwing in the towel. We want to give you hope. Life may be different now, but it is far from over. You may not be able to do the things you once did, but there are many new things to experience ahead of you. Fibromyalgia may affect your mind, body, and emotions, *but it does not define you*. It does not make you a lesser person. It does not get to dictate who you can become. It is not your mouthpiece or your judge. Fibro is an affliction, but it is not your commander. You can beat this! You can live a productive and rewarding life. I believe this with every fiber of my being.

You are loved.

If you would like to know more about our story, or would like to know more about what gives us real hope, please contact me at **mikeholien@me.com**.

We're all in this together,

Mike Holien

"Keep a goin'."

~Cecil Cook

FOLLOW UP

Since my article, Loving Those With Fibro has posted on my blog, I have had many people contact me with their stories of brokenness and pain. What I have learned is that there are many people who know what April and I are going through and can relate to the daily struggles we face. Even as I write this my wife is coming off of a terrible flare up that put our whole family life into a tale-spin, but, we are still kicking, and believe that today is going to be a great one, for her and for all of us. The one thing that many people have reiterated to me over and over is that they came to the realization that they are not alone in this, and for that I thank God. We are not alone. We have each other. I want to say that if you are a family member/pal of a Fibro friend, and you are feeling isolated and lonely, please find some people in your life who can speak life into you. I realize that caring for others can be exhausting. There was a time in my life when I struggled with "compassion fatigue", where I just could not hear about or help yet another sick person. I was at the end of my rope emotionally. If you find yourself there, please know I have been there and I get it. You need to take care that this disease does not rob you of your strength for life. Find a support group of people who understand your struggles. Make sure you take time to recharge yourself physically, emotionally and spiritually. If you are burned out, you CANNOT care for anyone. So take care not to burn out. Today I took my kids to school late, because I desperately needed the sleep. We live in a society that may say this is wrong, but my children missing 2 hrs. of school will not derail their education, and it meant everything to an exhausted husband and father.

Lastly… I have not really shared the spiritual side of our lives much. Not because we are ashamed or afraid to offend anyone, but out of respect for the many people who hold their spirituality private and personal, but it would be remiss to not mention it at all. As Christians, April and I have put our faith and hope in Jesus Christ. (Many people reject this because, "how could a loving God allow us to feel soooooooo crummy"?) But we say it is Jesus that has gotten us through thus far. We know it is through His strength that we face the next day with courage and joy. If you are interested in knowing more about this part of our journey please email me. We always look forward to honest and respectful dialog.

Once again, you are loved. Whether your are a Fibro sufferer or a Fibro friend, keep your head up. Keep smiling. Keep believing for better days. Kick Fibro's butt!

You Rock.

~M.

ACKNOWLEDGMENTS

-To the Via Media Group: Thank you for beta reading my work and spurring me on toward excellence.

-Peter Epler: Graphic Design Extraordinaire. You amaze me.

-Anne Bruce, thank you so much for contributing your editing skills. The time you put in is appreciated greatly. You are a blessing.

-Stacy Ihlenfeld: Your Fibro Pain Art is compelling. Thank you for helping others understand this disease through your beautiful talent. Thank you for allowing me to use your work.
http://smihlenfeld.wordpress.com

-Kristen Proby: Not only are you a successful writer, talented photographer, and wonderful sister; you're also a great friend. Thank you.

-Cliff Purcell: Thank you for challenging me to be a better writer. Thank you for your friendship. S.

REFERENCES

*http://www.niams.nih.gov/Health_Info/Fibromy
algia/fibromyalgia_ff.asp

Printed in Great Britain
by Amazon